METABOLIC CONFUSION DIET COOKBOOK FOR BEGINNERS TO PRO

Explore a collection of 1500 days' worth of delicious and metabolism-boosting recipes, accompanied by a 30-day meal plan designed to optimize your endomorph nutrition.

Vincent John Walker

DISCLAIMER

This publication is designed to provide competent and reliable information regarding the subject covered. However, the views expressed in this publication are those of the author alone, and should not be taken as expert instruction or professional advice. The reader is responsible for his or her actions. The author hereby disclaims any responsibility or liability whatsoever that is incurred from the use or application of the contents of this publication by the purchaser of the reader. The purchaser or reader is hereby responsible for his or her actions.

Table of Contents

INTRODUCTION

Unveiling the Metabolic Confusion Philosophy

Discover the essence of the Metabolic Confusion Diet, a philosophy that rejects one-size-fits-all solutions. This cookbook is your guide to unraveling the science behind metabolic confusion, empowering you to make informed dietary choices. Dive into the dynamic interplay of nutrients, meal timing, and food variety, allowing your body to adapt and optimize its metabolic processes.

Nourishing Your Body, Delighting Your Palate

Explore a rich collection of recipes that not only align with the principles of metabolic confusion but also celebrate the joy of eating. From vibrant salads to hearty mains and indulgent desserts, each recipe showcases the idea that healthy eating can be both delicious and fulfilling. Whether you're a kitchen novice or an experienced home cook, there's a culinary delight awaiting you on every page.

Your Culinary Guide

Navigate the culinary landscape with confidence using the cookbook's detailed guide. We've demystified the essentials, ensuring that even those new to the kitchen can effortlessly create flavorful and nutritious meals. Learn about key ingredients that form the foundation of metabolic confusion-friendly dishes and gain insights into cooking techniques that maximize the benefits of this dietary approach.

Tailored for Every Lifestyle

This cookbook caters to the diverse needs of our readers, offering a range of recipes tailored to various lifestyles. Whether you're a parent juggling family responsibilities, a fitness enthusiast seeking performance-oriented meals, or someone with specific dietary needs, find recipes that match your unique requirements. Busy schedules, dietary preferences, and culinary expertise are all taken into account.

Transforming Your Relationship with Food

Beyond a mere collection of recipes, this cookbook invites you to reshape your relationship with food. Embrace a positive and mindful approach to eating, recognizing that each meal is an opportunity to nourish your body and delight your senses. Bid farewell to restrictive diets and welcome a lifestyle that fosters a balanced and sustainable connection with food.

Your Culinary and Wellness Companion

Embark on a culinary adventure with the "Metabolic Confusion Diet Cookbook for Starters to Pro" and consider it more than just a book. It's your culinary and wellness companion, guiding you through the intricacies of metabolic confusion with practical advice, tantalizing recipes, and a wealth of information supporting your health journey.

The Culmination of Flavor and Well-Being

This cookbook goes beyond cooking; it's about creating meals that nourish both body and soul. Let its pages inspire, motivate, and guide you as you embrace the transformative power of the Metabolic Confusion Diet. Your journey to optimal health and culinary delight begins now!

METABOLIC CONFUSION BREAKFAST RECIPES

Avocado Toast

Ingredients:

- 2 slices of whole-grain bread
- 1 ripe avocado
- Salt and pepper to taste
- Red pepper flakes (optional)
- A drizzle of olive oil

Instructions:

- The pieces of bread should be toasted until they reach a crispiness.
- To prepare the avocado, split it in half lengthwise and remove the pit while the bread is being toasted. Take the meat and place it in a basin. Using a fork, mash the flesh.
- After the bread pieces have been toasted, spread the mashed avocado on them.
- Add some salt, pepper, and crushed red pepper flakes for seasoning (if desired).
- To finish, sprinkle some olive oil over the dish.

Nutritional Value (per serving):

- Calories: 260

- Protein: 7g

- Carbohydrates: 21g

- Fiber: 10g

- Healthy fats: 13g

Greek Yogurt Parfait

Ingredients:

- 1 cup Greek yogurt

- 1/2 cup fresh berries (e.g., strawberries, blueberries)

- 1/4 cup granola

- Honey (optional)

Instructions:

- First, layer the Greek yogurt, then the fresh berries, and finally the granola in a dish or glass.

- To add sweetness, honey may be drizzled on top, if preferred.

Nutritional Value (per serving):

- Calories: 303

- Protein: 13g

- Carbohydrates: 44g

- Fiber: 7g

- Healthy fats: 7g

Veggie Omelette

Ingredients:

- 2 large eggs
- 1/4 cup diced bell peppers
- 1/4 cup diced onions
- 1/4 cup diced tomatoes
- Salt and pepper to taste
- Cooking spray or a small amount of olive oil

Instructions:

- Salt and pepper should be added to the eggs after they have been whisked in a bowl.
- Coat a non-stick skillet with cooking spray or a little bit of olive oil and heat it over medium heat. The pan should go through this process.
- In a pan, add the diced veggies and sauté them until they reach the desired level of tenderness.
- After pouring the eggs that have been whisked over the vegetables, fry them for about two to three minutes on each side.

Nutritional Value (per serving):

- Calories: 222
- Protein: 15g
- Carbohydrates: 12g

- Fiber: 3g

- Healthy fats: 15g

Peanut Butter Banana Smoothie

Ingredients:

- 1 ripe banana

- 2 tablespoons peanut butter

- 1 cup almond milk (or any milk of your choice)

- 1/2 cup Greek yogurt

- 1 tablespoon honey (optional)

- Ice cubes

Instructions:

- Blend all of the ingredients in a blender.

- Blend until it is completely smooth.

- If you want your smoothie to be more thick, add more ice cubes.

Nutritional Value (per serving):

- Calories: 352

- Protein: 16g

- Carbohydrates: 42g

- Fiber: 7g

- Healthy fats: 16g

Overnight Chia Seed Pudding

Ingredients:

- 3 tablespoons chia seeds
- 1 cup almond milk (or any milk of your choice)
- 1/2 teaspoon vanilla extract
- Fresh berries for topping
- Honey (optional)

Instructions:

- Combining chia seeds, almond milk, and vanilla essence in a dish is the first step.
- Cover and place in the refrigerator for the night.
- First thing in the morning, garnish with some fresh berries and, if you so wish, a drizzle of honey.

Nutritional Value (per serving):

- Calories: 212
- Protein: 8g
- Carbohydrates: 23g
- Fiber: 14g
- Healthy fats: 11g

Spinach and Feta Breakfast Quesadilla

Ingredients:

- 2 whole-wheat tortillas
- 2 large eggs
- 1 cup fresh spinach leaves
- 1/4 cup crumbled feta cheese
- Salt and pepper to taste
- Cooking spray or a small amount of olive oil

Instructions:

- The spinach should be cooked in a skillet that does not adhere to the pan over medium heat until it wilts.
- Salt and pepper should be added to the eggs after they have been whisked in a separate bowl.
- One more skillet should be heated, and then it should be coated with cooking spray or a tiny bit of olive oil.
- After the eggs have been whisked, pour them into the pan and continue to cook them until they are set.
- The tortillas should be laid out, and then the scrambled eggs, spinach that has been sautéed, and feta cheese should be put on one side of each tortilla. They are folded in half.
- Heat in the skillet until the cheese is melted and both sides have a golden brown color.

Nutritional Value (per serving):

- Calories: 352
- Protein: 19g
- Carbohydrates: 26g
- Fiber: 8g
- Healthy fats: 16g

Banana Nut Oatmeal

Ingredients:

- 1/2 cup rolled oats
- 1 cup water or milk (of your choice)
- 1 ripe banana, sliced
- 1 tablespoon chopped nuts (e.g., walnuts or almonds)
- Cinnamon and honey (optional)

Instructions:

- It is necessary to bring the water or milk to a boil in a pot.
- To make the rolled oats creamy, add them and simmer them over medium heat for approximately five to seven minutes.
- After extra two minutes of cooking, stir in the sliced banana and continue to simmer.
- A sprinkling of cinnamon and chopped nuts should be sprinkled on top. Honey may be added if desired.

Nutritional Value (per serving):

- Calories: 355

- Protein: 10g

- Carbohydrates: 62g

- Fiber: 9g

- Healthy fats: 9g

Breakfast Burrito

Ingredients:

- 2 large eggs

- 1/4 cup black beans, drained and rinsed

- 1/4 cup diced bell peppers

- 1/4 cup diced onions

- 2 tablespoons shredded cheddar cheese

- Salt and pepper to taste

- Whole-wheat tortilla

Instructions:

- Salt and pepper should be added to the eggs after they have been whisked in a bowl.

- Coat a non-stick skillet with cooking spray or a little bit of olive oil and heat it over medium heat. The pan should go through this process.

- Add the veggies that have been diced and sauté them until they are tender.

- After whisking the eggs, pour them into the pan and scramble them until they are done.

- The tortilla made with whole wheat may be warmed in a separate pan or the microwave.

- When you are ready, place the cheese, scrambled eggs, and black beans inside the tortilla. Fold, and then take pleasure in it.

Nutritional Value (per serving):

- Calories: 352
- Protein: 17g
- Carbohydrates: 32g
- Fiber: 7g
- Healthy fats: 19g

Smoked Salmon and Cream Cheese Bagel

Ingredients:

- 1whole-grain or everything bagel
- 2 tablespoons low-fat cream cheese
- 2-3 slices of smoked salmon
- Sliced cucumber and red onion (optional)
- Fresh dill (optional)

Instructions:

- Toast the bagel after slicing it in half lengthwise.
- On each side of the bagel, spread cream cheese in a thin layer.
- Smoked salmon should be layered on top, and cucumber, red onion, and fresh dill may be added if desired too.
- Put the bagel halves together, and then savor them.

Nutritional Value (per serving):

- Calories: 299
- Protein: 16g
- Carbohydrates: 44g
- Fiber: 7g
- Healthy fats: 11g

Blueberry Pancakes

Ingredients:

- 1 cup whole-wheat pancake mix
- 1/2 cup fresh blueberries
- 1/2 cup almond milk (or any milk of your choice)
- 1 large egg
- Maple syrup (optional)

Instructions:

- Mix the pancake mix, almond milk, and egg in a basin that is suitable for mixing. Combine until it is completely smooth.
- Gently incorporate the fresh blueberries.
- A griddle or a skillet that does not stick should be heated at medium-high heat. To make each pancake, pour a quarter cup of batter onto the griddle.
- Once bubbles appear on the surface, turn the food and continue cooking until it reaches a golden brown color.
- Depending on your preference, serve with a sprinkle of maple syrup.

Nutritional Value (per serving):

- Calories: 303
- Protein: 12g
- Carbohydrates: 54g
- Fiber: 7g
- Healthy fats: 8g

Spinach and Mushroom Breakfast Quiche

Ingredients:

- 4 large eggs
- 1 cup fresh spinach, chopped

- 1/2 cup mushrooms, sliced
- 1/4 cup shredded mozzarella cheese
- Salt and pepper to taste

Instructions:

- Preheat the oven to 175 degrees Celsius (350 degrees Fahrenheit).
- Salt and pepper should be added to the eggs after they have been whisked in a bowl.
- Prepare the mushrooms by sautéing them in a pan that can go in the oven until they shed their moisture and become soft.
- Place the chopped spinach in the pan and continue to cook it until it has wilted.
- Pour the eggs that have been whisked over the vegetables, and then sprinkle the mozzarella cheese over top.
- If you want the quiche to be firm and gently browned, bake it for fifteen to twenty minutes.

Nutritional Value (per serving):

- Calories: 181
- Protein: 15g
- Carbohydrates: 4g
- Fiber: 2g
- Healthy fats: 10g

Breakfast Tacos

Ingredients:

- 2 small whole-wheat tortillas
- 2 large eggs, scrambled
- 1/4 cup black beans, drained and rinsed
- Salsa and sliced avocado for topping
- Salt and pepper to taste

Instructions:

- Prepare the tortillas by heating them in a microwave or a dry skillet.
- Put scrambled eggs, black beans, salsa, and sliced avocado on each tortilla. Fill each tortilla with the mixture.
- Use pepper and salt to season the food.
- The tortillas should be rolled up and enjoyed.

Nutritional Value (per serving):

- Calories: 322
- Protein: 17g
- Carbohydrates: 36g
- Fiber: 9g
- Healthy fats: 15g

Veggie Breakfast Hash

Ingredients:

- 2 large eggs
- 1/2 cup diced sweet potatoes
- 1/4 cup diced bell peppers
- 1/4 cup diced onions
- 1/4 cup diced zucchini
- Salt and pepper to taste
- Cooking spray or a small amount of olive oil

Instructions:

- Prepare the cooking spray or olive oil by heating it in a pan over medium heat.
- Cook the sweet potatoes for around five minutes, or until they begin to become more tender.
- After adding the chopped vegetables, sauté them until they are nice and soft and have a light brown color.
- The vegetables should be moved to the side, and the eggs should be broken into the pan. Strive to cook them by scrambling them.
- The eggs and vegetables should be combined, and then seasoned with salt and pepper before being served.

Nutritional Value (per serving):

- Calories: 263
- Protein: 14g
- Carbohydrates: 25g
- Fiber: 6g
- Healthy fats: 13g

Peanut Butter and Banana Overnight Oats

Ingredients:

- Half a cup of rolled oats
- One cup of almond milk (or any milk of your choice)
- one mashed, ripe banana
- Two tsp of peanut butter
- One tsp honey (optional)
- Crushed peanuts and sliced banana as a garnish

Instructions:

- Put the rolled oats, almond milk, mashed banana, and peanut butter into a bowl or jar and mix this mixture. Give it a good stir.
- If you so wish, drizzle honey over the top.
- Cover and place in the refrigerator for the night.
- On top, sprinkle some crushed peanuts and sliced bananas first thing in the morning.

Nutritional Value (per serving):

- Calories: 382
- Protein: 10g
- Carbohydrates: 53g
- Fiber: 9g
- Healthy fats: 14g

Breakfast Burrito Bowl

Ingredients:

- 1/2 cup cooked quinoa
- 1/4 cup black beans, drained and rinsed
- 1/4 cup diced tomatoes
- 1/4 cup diced avocado
- 1 large egg, fried or scrambled
- Salsa and chopped cilantro for topping
- Salt and pepper to taste

Instructions:

- Arrange the quinoa that has been cooked, the black beans, the chopped tomatoes, and the diced avocado in a bowl.
- A fried or scrambled egg should be placed on top.
- Use pepper and salt to season the food.
- Add some chopped cilantro and salsa to finish it off.

Nutritional Value (per serving):

- Calories: 381

- Protein: 15g

- Carbohydrates: 41g

- Fiber: 12g

- Healthy fats: 15g

Banana and Blueberry Protein Pancakes

Ingredients:

- 1 ripe banana, mashed

- 2 large eggs

- 1/4 cup rolled oats

- 1/4 cup blueberries

- 1/2 teaspoon vanilla extract

- Cooking spray or a small amount of olive oil

Instructions:

- Mix the mashed banana, eggs, rolled oats, and vanilla essence in a bowl until everything is well incorporated.

- Blueberries should be folded in well.

- Coat a non-stick skillet with cooking spray or a little bit of olive oil and heat it over medium heat. The pan should go through this process.

- To make each pancake, pour a quarter cup of batter onto the griddle.

- Once bubbles appear on the surface, turn the food and continue cooking until it reaches a golden brown color.

Nutritional Value (per serving):

- Calories: 322

- Protein: 16g

- Carbohydrates: 42g

- Fiber: 7g

- Healthy fats: 13g

Breakfast Quinoa Bowl

Ingredients:

- 1 cup cooked quinoa

- 1/4 cup Greek yogurt

- 1/4 cup mixed berries (e.g., strawberries, blueberries)

- 1 tablespoon honey

- Chopped nuts (e.g., almonds, walnuts) for topping

Instructions:

- Layer quinoa that has been cooked, Greek yogurt, and a variety of berries in a dish.

- Drip with honey and serve.

- Sprinkle some chopped nuts on top for an additional crunch and taste.

Nutritional Value (per serving):

- Calories: 352
- Protein: 12g
- Carbohydrates: 64g
- Fiber: 9g
- Healthy fats: 8g

Breakfast Tofu Scramble

Ingredients:

- 1/2 block of firm tofu, crumbled
- 1/4 cup diced bell peppers
- 1/4 cup diced onions
- 1/4 cup spinach leaves
- 1/2 teaspoon turmeric (for color)
- Salt and pepper to taste
- Cooking spray or a small amount of olive oil

Instructions:

- Coat a non-stick skillet with cooking spray or a little bit of olive oil and heat it over medium heat. The pan should go through this process.

- Sauté the chopped onions and bell peppers until they get as tender as possible.

- After adding the crushed tofu and turmeric, stir the mixture periodically until it is completely cooked.

- Cook the spinach until it has wilted, then toss it in.

- Sprinkle some salt and pepper on top, and then serve.

Nutritional Value (per serving):

- Calories: 242

- Protein: 17g

- Carbohydrates: 13g

- Fiber: 5g

- Healthy fats: 15g

Mango and Coconut Chia Pudding

Ingredients:

- 3 tablespoons chia seeds

- 1 cup coconut milk

- 1/2 cup diced mango

- 1 tablespoon shredded coconut

- 1 teaspoon honey (optional)

Instructions:

- Chia seeds and coconut milk should be mixed in a container or dish.

- Give it a good stir.

- To the mixture, add shredded coconut and chopped mango. Mix.

- For added sweetness, honey may be drizzled over top, if preferred.

- Refrigerate the mixture for a few hours or overnight with the lid on.

Nutritional Value (per serving):

- Calories: 322

- Protein: 6g

- Carbohydrates: 28g

- Fiber: 7g

- Healthy fats: 23g

Breakfast Berry Smoothie Bowl

Ingredients:

- 1 cup frozen mixed berries

- 1/2 ripe banana

- 1/2 cup Greek yogurt

- 1/4 cup granola

- Honey for drizzling (optional)

Instructions:

- A smooth consistency should be achieved by blending frozen berries, bananas, and Greek yogurt in a blender.
- The smoothie should be poured into a bowl.
- Granola may be sprinkled on top for a crunch, and honey can be drizzled on top if desired.

Nutritional Value (per serving):

- Calories: 287
- Protein: 16g
- Carbohydrates: 57g
- Fiber: 9g
- Healthy fats: 4g

LUNCH RECIPES

Grilled Chicken Salad

Ingredients:

- 4 oz (113g) grilled chicken breast, sliced
- 2 cups mixed greens (e.g., lettuce, spinach)
- 1/4 cup cherry tomatoes, halved
- 1/4 cup cucumber slices
- 2 tablespoons balsamic vinaigrette dressing

Instructions:

- Put the greens in a salad dish and toss them together.
- Incorporate the grilled chicken that has been cut, cherry tomatoes, and cucumber.
- Toss the salad gently after drizzling it with balsamic vinaigrette dressing.

Nutritional Value (per serving):

- Calories: 283
- Protein: 33g
- Carbohydrates: 3g
- Fiber: 4g
- Healthy fats: 15g

Quinoa and Black Bean Bowl

Ingredients:

- 1/2 cup cooked quinoa
- 1/2 cup black beans, drained and rinsed
- 1/4 cup diced red bell pepper
- 1/4 cup diced red onion
- 1/4 cup corn kernels
- 1/4 cup diced avocado Lime vinaigrette dressing

Instructions:

- Quinoa that has been cooked, black beans, red bell pepper, red onion, and corn should all be mixed in a dish.
- The lime vinaigrette dressing should be drizzled on top.
- As a garnish, add cubed avocado.

Nutritional Value (per serving):

- Calories: 342
- Protein: 12g
- Carbohydrates: 53g
- Fiber: 11g
- Healthy fats: 11g

Lentil and Vegetable Soup

Ingredients:

- 1 cup cooked lentils

- 1 cup mixed vegetables (e.g., carrots, celery, zucchini)

- 1/4 cup diced onion

- 2 cloves garlic, minced

- 4 cups vegetable broth

- 1 teaspoon dried thyme Salt and pepper to taste

Instructions:

- Sauté the chopped onion and garlic in a saucepan until the aroma is released.

- Include lentils, a variety of veggies, vegetable broth, and thyme in the dish.

- Use pepper and salt to season the food.

- Simmer for twenty to twenty-five minutes, or until the veggies are soft.

Nutritional Value (per serving):

- Calories: 260

- Protein: 19g

- Carbohydrates: 52g

- Fiber: 18g

- Healthy fats: 1g

Caprese Sandwich

Ingredients:

- 2 slices whole-grain bread

- 2 slices fresh mozzarella cheese

- 1 ripe tomato, sliced

- Fresh basil leaves

- Balsamic glaze

- Olive oil (optional)

Instructions:

- Olive oil may be drizzled on one side of each bread slice, although this step is optional.

- On one slice, layer mozzarella, tomato slices, and fresh basil. Repeat with the other slice.

- Apply a glaze made of balsamic vinegar.

- To finish, place the second piece of bread on top, oil-side down.

- You may either grill or press the cheese until it melts and the bread becomes toasted.

Nutritional Value (per serving):

- Calories: 323

- Protein: 14g

- Carbohydrates: 32g

- Fiber: 5g

- Healthy fats: 12g

Teriyaki Tofu Stir-Fry

Ingredients:

- 1 cup cubed tofu
- cup broccoli florets
- 1/2 cup sliced bell peppers
- 1/2 cup sliced carrots
- tablespoons teriyaki sauce
- 1 tablespoon sesame oil
- Cooked brown rice

Instructions:

- In a pan, heat the sesame oil over medium-high heat.
- Add the tofu cubes and stir-fry until gently browned.
- Combine broccoli, bell peppers, and carrots. Stir and cook till tender.
- Add the teriyaki sauce to the stir-fry and heat for another minute.
- Serve with cooked brown rice.

Nutritional Value (per serving):

- Calories: 370
- Protein: 15g
- Carbohydrates: 33g
- Fiber: 5g

- Healthy fats: 17g

Mediterranean Chickpea Salad

Ingredients:

- 1 cup canned chickpeas, drained and rinsed
- 1/2 cucumber, diced
- 1/2 cup cherry tomatoes, halved
- 1/4 cup red onion, finely chopped
- 1/4 cup feta cheese, crumbled
- Kalamata olives (optional)
- Greek dressing

Instructions:

- In a mixing bowl, add chickpeas, cucumber, cherry tomatoes, and red onion.
- If preferred, mix with crumbled feta cheese and Kalamata olives.
- Drizzle with Greek dressing and mix.

Nutritional Value (per serving):

- Calories: 322
- Protein: 13g
- Carbohydrates: 33g
- Fiber: 8g
- Healthy fats: 13g

Turkey and Avocado Wrap

Ingredients:

- 1 whole-grain wrap
- 3 oz (85g) sliced turkey breast
- 1/4 avocado, sliced
- Lettuce leaves
- Tomato slices
- Mustard or mayo (optional)

Instructions:

- Lay the whole-grain wrap flat.
- Layer with turkey slices, avocado, lettuce, and tomato.
- If desired, season with mustard or mayonnaise.
- Roll up the wrap and cut it in half.

Nutritional Value (per serving):

- Calories: 322
- Protein: 23g
- Carbohydrates: 34g
- Fiber: 8g
- Healthy fats: 15g

Spaghetti Aglio e Olio with Broccoli

Ingredients:

- 2 oz (56g) whole-wheat spaghetti

- 1/2 cup broccoli florets

- 2 cloves garlic, minced

- 2 tablespoons olive oil

- Red pepper flakes (optional)

- Grated Parmesan cheese

Instructions:

- Cook the spaghetti according to package directions, adding the broccoli for the final 2 minutes.

- In a pan, heat the olive oil over medium heat. If preferred, season with minced garlic and red pepper flakes.

- Toss cooked spaghetti and broccoli in a pan with garlic oil.

- Start serving with grated Parmesan cheese.

Nutritional Value (per serving):

- Calories: 353

- Protein: 11g

- Carbohydrates: 54g

- Fiber: 9g

- Healthy fats: 12g

BBQ Chickpea and Veggie Bowl

Ingredients:

- 1 cup canned chickpeas, drained and rinsed

- 1/2 cup diced bell peppers
- 1/2 cup diced red onion
- 1/2 cup corn kernels
- 2 tablespoons BBQ sauce
- Cooked brown rice

Instructions:

- In a pan, cook the diced bell peppers and red onion until tender.
- Combine the chickpeas and corn, then whisk in the BBQ sauce.
- Serve with cooked brown rice.

Nutritional Value (per serving):

- Calories: 346
- Protein: 15g
- Carbohydrates: 64g
- Fiber: 13g
- Healthy fats: 7g

Caprese Quinoa Salad

Ingredients:

- 1 cup cooked quinoa
- 1 cup cherry tomatoes, halved
- 1/2 cup fresh mozzarella balls

- Fresh basil leaves
- Balsamic glaze
- Olive oil (optional)

Instructions:

- In a bowl, mix cooked quinoa, cherry tomatoes, and fresh mozzarella balls.
- Add fresh basil leaves.
- Drizzle with balsamic glaze and olive oil, if preferred.

Nutritional Value (per serving):

- Calories: 310
- Protein: 11g
- Carbohydrates: 36g
- Fiber: 5g
- Healthy fats: 17g

Tuna Salad Lettuce Wraps

Ingredients:

- 1 can (5 oz) tuna in water, drained
- 2 tablespoons Greek yogurt (or mayonnaise)
- 1/4 cup diced celery
- 1/4 cup diced red onion
- 1 teaspoon Dijon mustard
- Lettuce leaves for wrapping

- Sliced avocado (optional)

Instructions:

- In a mixing dish, add tuna, Greek yogurt, chopped celery, diced red onion, and Dijon mustard.
- Spoon tuna salad onto lettuce leaves.
- If desired, add some sliced avocado.
- Wrap, and enjoy!

Nutritional Value (per serving):

- Calories: 222
- Protein: 23g
- Carbohydrates: 7g
- Fiber: 3g
- Healthy fats: 8g

Vegetable and Hummus Wrap

Ingredients:

- 1 whole-grain wrap
- 2 tablespoons hummus
- Sliced cucumber
- Sliced bell peppers
- Shredded carrots
- Leafy greens

Instructions:

- The whole-grain wrap should be covered with hummus in an equal layer.
- Incorporate shredded carrots, sliced cucumbers, bell peppers, and leafy greens into the mixture.
- Wrap the wrap in a roll, then cut it in half.

Nutritional Value (per serving):

- Calories: 270
- Protein: 9g
- Carbohydrates: 42g
- Fiber: 11g
- Healthy fats: 10g

Chicken and Vegetable Stir-Fry

Ingredients:

- 4 oz (113g) cooked chicken breast, sliced
- 1 cup mixed vegetables (e.g., broccoli, bell peppers, snap peas)
- 2 cloves garlic, minced
- 2 tablespoons low-sodium soy sauce
- 1 tablespoon sesame oil
- Cooked brown rice

Instructions:

- Make sure the sesame oil is heated up over medium-high heat in a wok or pan.
- Combine the chicken slices with the minced garlic. Stir-fry the chicken until it is completely comfortable.
- After adding the veggies, stir-fry them until they are soft.
- When the stir-fry is done, pour low-sodium soy sauce over it.
- On top of brown rice that has been cooked.

Nutritional Value (per serving):

- Calories: 332
- Protein: 27g
- Carbohydrates: 35g
- Fiber: 9g
- Healthy fats: 12g

Mediterranean Quinoa Bowl

Ingredients:

- 1 cup cooked quinoa
- 1/4 cup diced cucumbers
- 1/4 cup diced tomatoes
- 1/4 cup diced red onion
- 1/4 cup Kalamata olives, pitted and chopped

- Feta cheese crumbles

- Tzatziki sauce

Instructions:

- Quinoa that has been cooked through, diced cucumbers, diced tomatoes, diced red onion, and Kalamata olives should be mixed in a dish.

- Crumbled feta cheese should be sprinkled on top.

- Finish with a drizzle of tzatziki sauce.

Nutritional Value (per serving):

- Calories: 321

- Protein: 9g

- Carbohydrates: 40g

- Fiber: 8g

- Healthy fats: 11g

Thai Peanut Noodle Salad

Ingredients:

- 2 oz (56g) whole-wheat noodles

- 1/4 cup peanut sauce

- 1/2 cup shredded cabbage

- 1/4 cup shredded carrots

- 1/4 cup chopped scallions Crushed peanuts for topping

Instructions:

- The directions on the packaging should be followed while cooking whole-wheat noodles.
- Mix peanut sauce with noodles that have been cooked.
- Incorporate chopped onions, shredded cabbage, and shredded carrots into the mixture. Toss once more.
- Use crushed peanuts as a topping.

Nutritional Value (per serving):

- Calories: 365
- Protein: 15g
- Carbohydrates: 56g
- Fiber: 9g
- Healthy fats: 13g

Chickpea and Avocado Salad

Ingredients:

- 1 cup canned chickpeas, drained and rinsed
- 1/2 avocado, diced
- 1/4 cup diced red onion
- 1/4 cup diced cucumber
- 1/4 cup diced red bell pepper
- Fresh cilantro (or parsley) for garnish

- Lemon vinaigrette dressing

Instructions:

- Combine the chickpeas, avocado, red onion, cucumber, and red bell pepper in a bowl by mixing them.
- Add a dressing made with lemon vinaigrette and drizzle.
- Fresh cilantro or parsley may be used as a decorator.

Nutritional Value (per serving):

- Calories: 336
- Protein: 8g
- Carbohydrates: 33g
- Fiber: 12g
- Healthy fats: 11g

Turkey and Quinoa Stuffed Bell Peppers

Ingredients:

- 2 bell peppers, halved and seeded
- 1/2 cup cooked quinoa
- 4 oz (113g) ground turkey
- 1/4 cup diced tomatoes
- 1/4 cup diced onions
- 1/4 cup shredded cheddar cheese (optional)
- Taco seasoning
- Salsa for topping

Instructions:

- Preheat the oven to 175 degrees Celsius (350 degrees Fahrenheit).
- After browning the ground turkey in a pan, add taco spice to the mixture.
- Quinoa that has been cooked, diced tomatoes, and diced onions should be combined in the pan.
- The turkey-quinoa mixture should be stuffed into each side of the bell pepper.
- If you so wish, sprinkle some shredded cheddar cheese on top.
- Peppers should be baked for 25 to 30 minutes, or until they are soft.
- Serve with salsa on the side.

Nutritional Value (per serving, 2 halves):

- Calories: 352
- Protein: 25g
- Carbohydrates: 32g
- Fiber: 7g
- Healthy fats: 14g

Pesto Pasta Salad with Cherry Tomatoes

Ingredients:

- 2 oz (56g) whole-wheat pasta
- 1/4 cup cherry tomatoes, halved
- 2 tablespoons pesto sauce
- Fresh basil leaves for garnish
- Parmesan cheese (optional)

Instructions:

- Prepare pasta made with whole wheat while following the directions on the box.
- Toss the pasta that has been cooked with the pesto sauce and cherry tomatoes.
- If you so wish, garnish with fresh basil leaves and Parmesan cheese.

Nutritional Value (per serving):

- Calories: 332
- Protein: 9g
- Carbohydrates: 43g
- Fiber: 6g
- Healthy fats: 13g

Egg and Spinach Wrap

Ingredients:

- 2 large eggs, scrambled

- 1 cup fresh spinach leaves

- 1 whole-grain wrap

- Salsa (optional)

- Sliced avocado (optional)

Instructions:

- The eggs should be scrambled in a pan until they are done.

- On a wrap made with whole grains, arrange some fresh spinach leaves.

- Include eggs that have been scrambled.

- If you so wish, stir in some salsa and sliced avocado.

- To serve, roll up the wrap.

Nutritional Value (per serving):

- Calories: 293

- Protein: 17g

- Carbohydrates: 23g

- Fiber: 13g

- Healthy fats: 13g

Vegetarian Sushi Rolls

Ingredients:

- Nori seaweed sheets

- 1 cup cooked sushi rice

- Sliced cucumber

- Sliced avocado
- Carrot matchsticks

Instructions:

- A dipping sauce consisting of pickled ginger and low-sodium soy sauce
- You should lay a bamboo sushi rolling mat down on a clean surface.
- The mat should be covered with a layer of plastic wrap. The plastic wrap should be covered with a layer of nori.
- On top of the nori, spread sushi rice in a uniform layer, leaving a thin border at the top.
- Matchsticks of carrots, cucumbers, and avocados should be added.
- Through the use of the bamboo mat and the application of little pressure, roll up the sushi.
- The pickled ginger and soy sauce should be served with bite-sized pieces that have been sliced.

Nutritional Value (per serving):

- Calories: 302
- Protein: 7g
- Carbohydrates: 63g
- Fiber: 7g
- Healthy fats: 7g

Minestrone Soup

Ingredients:

- 1 cup cooked pasta (e.g., small shells)
- 1/2 cup canned kidney beans, drained and rinsed
- 1/2 cup diced tomatoes
- 1/4 cup diced carrots
- 1/4 cup diced celery
- 1/4 cup diced zucchini
- 4 cups vegetable broth
- 1 teaspoon Italian seasoning
- Grated Parmesan cheese (optional)

Instructions:

- Put the pasta that has been prepared, kidney beans, chopped tomatoes, carrots, celery, and zucchini into a saucepan and start cooking.
- Stir in with Italian spice, then pour in some veggie broth.
- For fifteen to twenty minutes, simmer the veggies until they are soft.
- Depending on your preference, serve with grated Parmesan cheese.

Nutritional Value (per serving):

- Calories: 282
- Protein: 13g

- Carbohydrates: 52g
- Fiber: 9g
- Healthy fats: 4g

Shrimp and Asparagus Stir-Fry

Ingredients:

- 4 oz (113g) shrimp, peeled and deveined
- 1 cup asparagus spears, trimmed and cut into 2-inch pieces
- 1/4 cup sliced bell peppers
- 2 cloves garlic, minced
- 1 tablespoon low-sodium soy sauce
- 1 tablespoon sesame oil
- Cooked brown rice

Instructions:

- Make sure the sesame oil is heated up in a pan over medium-high heat.
- Garlic that has been minced and shrimp should be added. Prepare the shrimp till they become pink.
- Stir-frying the asparagus and bell peppers until they are soft is the next step.
- When the stir-fry is done, pour low-sodium soy sauce over it.
- On top of brown rice that has been cooked.

Nutritional Value (per serving):

- Calories: 311
- Protein: 25g
- Carbohydrates: 34g
- Fiber: 7g
- Healthy fats: 11g

Black Bean and Corn Salad

Ingredients:

- 1 cup canned black beans, drained and rinsed
- 1/2 cup corn kernels (fresh, frozen, or canned)
- 1/4 cup diced red onion
- 1/4 cup diced bell peppers
- Lime vinaigrette dressing
- Fresh cilantro for garnish

Instructions:

- Black beans, corn, chopped red onion, and diced bell peppers should be mixed in a dish.
- The lime vinaigrette dressing should be drizzled on top.
- Serve with a garnish of fresh cilantro.

Nutritional Value (per serving):

- Calories: 282

- Protein: 13g

- Carbohydrates: 53g

- Fiber: 13g

- Healthy fats: 3g

Teriyaki Chicken and Broccoli

Ingredients:

- 4 oz (113g) cooked chicken breast, sliced

- 1 cup broccoli florets

- 2 tablespoons teriyaki sauce

- 1 teaspoon sesame seeds

- Cooked brown rice

Instructions:

- Broccoli should be stir-fried in a pan until it is soft.

- Include teriyaki sauce and chicken pieces that have been cooked. Turn the heat up.

- On top of brown rice that has been cooked.

- Sesame seeds are used as a garnish.

Nutritional Value (per serving):

- Calories: 322

- Protein: 30g

- Carbohydrates: 46g

- Fiber: 7g

- Healthy fats: 6g

Greek Chicken Wrap

Ingredients:

- 3 oz (85g) cooked chicken breast, sliced
- 1 whole-grain wrap
- 2 tablespoons tzatziki sauce
- Sliced cucumber
- Sliced red onion
- Sliced tomatoes
- Fresh spinach leaves

Instructions:

- Spread out the wrap made with healthy grains.
- On the wrap, spread the tzatziki sauce in a uniform layer.
- Chicken pieces, cucumber slices, red onion slices, tomato slices, and fresh spinach should be layered on top.
- Take the wrap and roll it up before cutting it in half.

Nutritional Value (per serving):

- Calories: 332
- Protein: 29g
- Carbohydrates: 32g

- Fiber: 8g
- Healthy fats: 12g

DINNER RECIPES

Grilled Lemon Herb Chicken

Ingredients:

- 4 boneless, skinless chicken breasts
- Zest and juice of 1 lemon
- 2 cloves garlic, minced
- 1 tablespoon fresh rosemary, minced
- 1 tablespoon fresh thyme, minced
- Salt and black pepper to taste
- Olive oil for grilling

Instructions:

- Garlic that has been minced, rosemary, thyme, salt, and black pepper should be combined with lemon zest and lemon juice in a bowl.
- First, place the chicken breasts in a plastic bag that can be sealed back up, and then pour the marinade over them.
- Seal the bag, and place it in the refrigerator for at least half an hour.
- Olive oil should be brushed over the grill once it has been preheated to medium-high heat.
- To ensure that the chicken is cooked through, grill it for around 6-7 minutes each side.

- The salad or veggies of your choice should be served alongside.

Nutritional Value (per serving):

- Calories: 231
- Protein: 42g
- Carbohydrates: 4g
- Fiber: 2g
- Healthy fats: 7g

Quinoa and Black Bean Stuffed Peppers

Ingredients:

- 4 bell peppers, tops removed and seeds removed
- 1 cup cooked quinoa
- 1 cup canned black beans, drained and rinsed
- 1 cup diced tomatoes
- 1/2 cup diced onions
- 1/2 cup shredded cheddar cheese (optional)
- Taco seasoning
- Salsa for topping

Instructions:

- Preheat the oven to 175 degrees Celsius (350 degrees Fahrenheit).

- Diced onions should be cooked in a pan until they become transparent.

- Quinoa that has been cooked, black beans, diced tomatoes, and taco spice should be added. Cook for three to five minutes.

- Prepare the bell peppers by stuffing them with a combination of quinoa and black beans.

- If you so wish, sprinkle some shredded cheddar cheese on top.

- Peppers should be baked for 25 to 30 minutes, or until they are soft.

- Serve with salsa on the side.

Nutritional Value (per serving, 1 stuffed pepper):

- Calories: 282
- Protein: 15g
- Carbohydrates: 41g
- Fiber: 10g
- Healthy fats: 8g

Baked Salmon with Lemon-Dill Sauce

Ingredients:

- 4 salmon fillets
- 2 tablespoons olive oil
- Zest and juice of 1 lemon

- 2 tablespoons fresh dill, chopped

- Salt and black pepper to taste

Instructions:

- Preheat the oven to 375 degrees Fahrenheit (190 degrees Celsius).

- Olive oil, lemon zest, lemon juice, chopped dill, salt, and black pepper should be combined in a small basin and stirred together.

- Salmon fillets should be placed on a baking pan that has been lined with parchment paper.

- Apply a thin layer of the lemon-dill mixture to the salmon fish.

- Salmon should be baked for fifteen to twenty minutes, or until it can be readily flaked with a fork.

- Serve with veggies that have been steamed or with a side salad.

Nutritional Value (per serving):

- Calories: 313

- Protein: 31g

- Carbohydrates: 5g

- Fiber: 0g

- Healthy fats: 21g

Veggie Stir-Fry with Tofu

Ingredients:

- 8 oz (226g) extra-firm tofu, cubed
- 2 cups mixed vegetables (e.g., bell peppers, broccoli, carrots)
- 1/4 cup low-sodium soy sauce
- 2 cloves garlic, minced
- 1 tablespoon ginger, minced
- 1 tablespoon sesame oil
- Cooked brown rice

Instructions:

- Make sure the sesame oil is heated up in a pan over medium-high heat.
- The cubed tofu should be cooked until it has a light brown color.
- Once the tofu has been removed from the pan, put it aside.
- Put the ginger and garlic that have been minced into the same skillet. Saute for one to two minutes.
- After adding the veggies, stir-fry them until they are soft.
- Once the tofu has been returned to the pan, add the low-sodium soy sauce.
- Two more minutes of cooking time are required.
- Serve with cooked brown rice.

Nutritional Value (per serving):

- Calories: 351

- Protein: 19g

- Carbohydrates: 32g

- Fiber: 7g

- Healthy fats: 15g

Mediterranean Chickpea Salad

Ingredients:

- 2 cups canned chickpeas, drained and rinsed

- 1 cup cucumber, diced

- 1 cup cherry tomatoes, halved

- 1/2 cup red onion, diced

- 1/4 cup Kalamata olives, pitted and sliced

- Feta cheese (optional)

- Greek dressing

Instructions:

- A mixture of chickpeas, cucumber, cherry tomatoes, red onion, and Kalamata olives should be mixed in a bowl.

- After drizzling with Greek dressing, stir the ingredients together.

- Crumbled feta cheese may be sprinkled on top if desired.

Nutritional Value (per serving):

- Calories: 262
- Protein: 11g
- Carbohydrates: 43g
- Fiber: 14g
- Healthy fats: 7g

Spaghetti Squash with Pesto and Cherry Tomatoes

Ingredients:

- 1 medium spaghetti squash
- 1 cup cherry tomatoes, halved
- 1/4 cup pesto sauce
- Grated Parmesan cheese (optional)
- Fresh basil leaves for garnish

Instructions:

- Preheat the oven to 375 degrees Fahrenheit (190 degrees Celsius).
- A longitudinal cut should be made in the spaghetti squash, and the seeds should be removed.
- The squash halves should be placed on a baking pan with the sliced side down.
- To ensure that the squash is soft, roast it for thirty to forty minutes.

- Using a fork, scrape the flesh to make strands that resemble spaghetti.

- Toss the strands of squash with the pesto sauce and cherry tomatoes then set aside.

- Put some grated Parmesan cheese and some fresh basil leaves on top as a garnish.

Nutritional Value (per serving):

- Calories: 222

- Protein: 5g

- Carbohydrates: 23g

- Fiber: 7g

- Healthy fats: 16g

Turkey and Vegetable Stir-Fry

Ingredients:

- 1 (450g) ground turkey

- 2 cups mixed vegetables (e.g., broccoli, bell peppers, snap peas)

- 1/4 cup low-sodium soy sauce

- 2 cloves garlic, minced

- 1 tablespoon ginger, minced

- 1 tablespoon sesame oil

- Cooked brown rice

Instructions:

- Make sure the sesame oil is heated up in a big pan over medium-high heat.
- After adding the ground turkey, heat it until it is browned, breaking it up with a spoon as it cooks.
- Take the turkey out of the skillet and store it in a separate location.
- Put the ginger and garlic that have been minced into the same skillet. Saute for one to two minutes.
- After adding the veggies, stir-fry them until they are soft.
- The turkey should be returned to the pan, and low-sodium soy sauce should be added. Two more minutes of cooking time are required.
- Serve with cooked brown rice.

Nutritional Value (per serving):

- Calories: 324
- Protein: 23g
- Carbohydrates: 23g
- Fiber: 6g
- Healthy fats: 13g

Spinach and Feta Stuffed Chicken Breasts

Ingredients:

- 4 boneless, skinless chicken breasts
- 1 cup fresh spinach leaves
- 1/2 cup crumbled feta cheese
- 1 clove garlic, minced
- 1 tablespoon olive oil Salt and black pepper to taste

Instructions:

- Preheat the oven to 375 degrees Fahrenheit (190 degrees Celsius).
- Prepare the olive oil by heating it in a pan over medium heat.
- Minced garlic and spinach should be added. Stir-fry the spinach until it wilts. After taking the dish off the heat, whisk in the crumbled feta cheese.
- A pocket should be cut into each chicken breast, and then the spinach and feta mixture should be stuffed into the pocket.
- Both salt and black pepper should be used to season the chicken breasts.
- Bake the chicken for twenty-five to thirty minutes, or until it is all the way done.

Nutritional Value (per serving):

- Calories: 281
- Protein: 42g

- Carbohydrates: 3g

- Fiber: 2g

- Healthy fats: 10g

Lentil and Vegetable Curry

Ingredients:

- 1 cup dried green or brown lentils

- 2 cups vegetable broth

- 1 cup diced tomatoes

- 1 cup mixed vegetables (e.g., bell peppers, carrots, peas)

- 1 onion, diced

- 2 cloves garlic, minced

- 1 tablespoon curry powder

- 1 tablespoon olive oil cooked quinoa or brown rice

Instructions:

- Prepare the olive oil by heating it in a large saucepan over medium heat.

- The onion and garlic should be diced. Sauté until the liquid becomes transparent.

- Curry powder should be stirred in and cooked for one minute.

- A mixture of lentils, diced tomatoes, vegetable broth, and mixed veggies should be added. Assume a boiling point.

- Lower the heat, cover the pot, and let it simmer for twenty to twenty-five minutes, or until the lentils and veggies are cooked.

- Serve on quinoa or brown rice that has been cooked.

Nutritional Value (per serving):

- Calories: 329

- Protein: 16g

- Carbohydrates: 53g

- Fiber: 16g

- Healthy fats: 6g

Shrimp and Broccoli Alfredo

Ingredients:

- 8 oz (226g) whole wheat fettuccine

- 1 lb (450g) shrimp, peeled and deveined

- 2cups broccoli florets

- 1 cup low-fat Alfredo sauce

- Grated Parmesan cheese for topping

- Fresh parsley for garnish

Instructions:

- Cook the fettuccine following the directions on the box. At the very end of the cooking process, add the broccoli vegetables. Drain.

- Cook the shrimp in a large pan over medium-high heat until they lose their pink color and become opaque.

- Put the fettuccine that has been cooked, the broccoli, and the Alfredo sauce into the pan. Mix everything and bring it to a boil.

- Cheese grated from Parmesan and fresh parsley should be served alongside.

Nutritional Value (per serving):

- Calories: 382
- Protein: 33g
- Carbohydrates: 42g
- Fiber: 7g
- Healthy fats: 10g

Baked Sweet Potato and Black Bean Tacos

Ingredients:

- 4 small sweet potatoes
- 1 can (15 oz) black beans, drained and rinsed
- 1 teaspoon chili powder
- 1/2 teaspoon cumin
- 8 small corn tortillas
- Salsa, avocado slices, and cilantro for topping

Instructions:

- Preheat the oven to 400 degrees Fahrenheit (200 degrees Celsius).

- After piercing sweet potatoes with a fork, bake them for forty-five to fifty minutes, or until they are soft.

- Put the black beans, chili powder, and cumin into a pot and mix them. Cook over a heat setting of medium until the food is completely heated.

- The sweet potatoes should be cut open, and the flesh should be fluffed with a fork.

- A sweet potato, black bean combination, and any toppings of your choosing should be placed into each tortilla.

Nutritional Value (per serving - 2 tacos):

- Calories: 320

- Protein: 11g

- Carbohydrates: 72g

- Fiber: 11g

- Healthy fats: 3g

Lemon Garlic Shrimp and Asparagus

Ingredients:

- 1 lb (450g) shrimp, peeled and deveined

- 1 bunch asparagus, trimmed

- Zest and juice of 1 lemon

- 2 cloves garlic, minced

- 2 tablespoons olive oil

- Salt and black pepper to taste

Instructions:

- Preheat the oven to 400 degrees Fahrenheit (200 degrees Celsius).

- Combine the lemon zest, lemon juice, minced garlic, olive oil, salt, and black pepper in a bowl and mix all of the ingredients.

- Mix the lemon-garlic mixture with the shrimp and asparagus, and toss to combine.

- Uniformly arrange them on a baking sheet.

- Roast for ten to twelve minutes, or until the shrimp are opaque and pink in color.

- Serve with quinoa or brown rice that has been cooked.

Nutritional Value (per serving):

- Calories: 272

- Protein: 31g

- Carbohydrates: 9g

- Fiber: 4g

- Healthy fats: 14g

Turkey and Vegetable Skillet

Ingredients:

- 1 lb (450g) ground turkey
- 2 cups mixed vegetables (e.g., bell peppers, zucchini, carrots)
- 1 onion, diced
- 2 cloves garlic, minced
- 1 tablespoon olive oil
- 1 tablespoon Italian seasoning
- Salt and black pepper to taste

Instructions:

- Prepare the olive oil by heating it in a large pan over medium-high heat.
- The onion and garlic should be diced. Sauté until the liquid becomes transparent.
- After adding the ground turkey, heat it until it is browned, breaking it up with a spoon as it cooks.
- Combine a variety of veggies, Italian seasoning, salt, and black pepper after stirring them in.
- Cook the turkey until it is completely cooked through and the veggies are soft.
- Whole wheat pasta may be served either "as is" or "overcooked."

Nutritional Value (per serving):

- Calories: 292
- Protein: 25g
- Carbohydrates: 13g
- Fiber: 5g
- Healthy fats: 17g

Portobello Mushroom and Spinach Stuffed Peppers

Ingredients:

- 4 bell peppers, tops removed and seeds removed
- 4 large portobello mushrooms, chopped
- 2 cups fresh spinach
- 1 cup cooked quinoa
- 1/2 cup shredded mozzarella cheese
- 2 cloves garlic, minced
- 1 tablespoon olive oil Salt and black pepper to taste

Instructions:

- Preheat the oven to 175 degrees Celsius (350 degrees Fahrenheit).
- Prepare the olive oil by heating it in a pan over medium heat.
- Include portobello mushrooms and garlic that have been minced. Sauté the mushrooms until they reach the desired tenderness.
- Add the fresh spinach and continue to cook until it has wilted.

- After removing the pan from the heat, include the quinoa that has been cooked, shredded mozzarella cheese, salt, and black pepper.
- Stuff the bell peppers with the mixture that consists of the mushrooms and spinach.
- Peppers should be baked for 25 to 30 minutes, or until they are soft.

Nutritional Value (per serving, 1 stuffed pepper):

- Calories: 262
- Protein: 12g
- Carbohydrates: 34g
- Fiber: 7g
- Healthy fats: 11g

Veggie and Tofu Stir-Fry

Ingredients:

- 8 oz (226g) extra-firm tofu, cubed
- 2 cups mixed vegetables (e.g., broccoli, bell peppers, snow peas)
- 1/4 cup low-sodium stir-fry sauce
- 1 tablespoon olive oil
- Cooked brown rice

Instructions:

- Prepare the olive oil by heating it in a pan over medium-high heat.

- The cubed tofu should be cooked until it has a light brown color.

- Once the tofu has been removed from the pan, put it aside.

- Stir-frying the veggies for three to five minutes in the same pan adds a variety of vegetables.

- Include low-sodium stir-fry sauce in the pan once the tofu has been returned to it. Two more minutes of cooking time are required.

- On top of brown rice that has been cooked.

Nutritional Value (per serving):

- Calories: 321
- Protein: 13g
- Carbohydrates: 45g
- Fiber: 7g
- Healthy fats: 14g

Teriyaki Chicken and Vegetable Stir-Fry

Ingredients:

- 1 lb (450g) boneless, skinless chicken breasts, cut into strips
- 2 cups mixed vegetables (e.g., broccoli, bell peppers, snap peas)
- 1/4 cup low-sodium teriyaki sauce

- 2 cloves garlic, minced
- 1 tablespoon ginger, minced
- 1 tablespoon sesame oil
- Cooked brown rice

Instructions:

- Make sure the sesame oil is heated up in a big pan over medium-high heat. Minced garlic and ginger should be added. Saute for one to two minutes.
- Place chicken strips in the pan and heat them until they are browned and cooked through.
- Once the chicken has been removed from the pan, put it aside.
- Add the veggies of your choice to the same pan and stir-fry them until they are cooked.
- Chicken should be returned to the pan, and low-sodium teriyaki sauce should be added. Two more minutes of cooking time are required.
- Serve over cooked brown rice.

Nutritional Value (per serving):

- Calories: 310
- Protein: 35g
- Carbohydrates: 43g
- Fiber: 9g

- Healthy fats: 8g

Lentil and Mushroom Stuffed Bell Peppers

Ingredients:

- 4 bell peppers, tops removed and seeds removed
- 1 cup brown lentils, cooked
- 1 cup mushrooms, chopped
- 1/2 cup diced tomatoes
- 1/2 cup diced onions
- 1/4 cup vegetable broth
- 1/4 cup shredded mozzarella cheese (optional)
- Italian seasoning
- Salt and black pepper to taste

Instructions:

- Preheat the oven to 175 degrees Celsius (350 degrees Fahrenheit).
- Prepare the mushrooms and onions by sautéing them in a pan until they are soft.
- The brown lentils that have been cooked, chopped tomatoes, Italian seasoning, salt, and black pepper should be stirred in. Cook for three to five minutes.
- Prepare the bell peppers by stuffing them with a combination of lentils and mushrooms.
- If you so wish, sprinkle some shredded mozzarella cheese on top.

- Peppers should be baked for 25 to 30 minutes, or until they are soft.

Nutritional Value (per serving, 1 stuffed pepper):

- Calories: 242

- Protein: 15g

- Carbohydrates: 42g

- Fiber: 11g

- Healthy fats: 3g

Beef and Broccoli Stir-Fry

Ingredients:

- 1 lb (450g) beef sirloin, thinly sliced

- 2 cups broccoli florets

- 1/4 cup low-sodium soy sauce

- 2 cloves garlic, minced

- 1 tablespoon ginger, minced

- 1 tablespoon olive oil

- Cooked brown rice

Instructions:

- Prepare the olive oil by heating it in a pan over medium-high heat.

- Minced garlic and ginger should be added. Saute for one to two minutes.

- Slices of meat should be added and fried until they are browned and cooked through.
- Once the steak has been removed from the pan, put it aside.
- You should add broccoli florets to the same pan and stir-fry them until they are cooked.
- Add the low-sodium soy sauce to the skillet and then return the steak to the pan.
- Two more minutes of cooking time are required.
- Serve over cooked brown rice.

Nutritional Value (per serving):

- Calories: 354
- Protein: 33g
- Carbohydrates: 29g
- Fiber: 7g
- Healthy fats: 13g

Caprese Stuffed Chicken

Ingredients:

- 4 boneless, skinless chicken breasts
- 1 cup cherry tomatoes, halved
- 1/2 cup fresh mozzarella cheese, diced
- 1/4 cup fresh basil leaves, chopped
- Balsamic glaze for drizzling
- Olive oil for cooking Salt and black pepper to taste

Instructions:

- Preheat the oven to 375 degrees Fahrenheit (190 degrees Celsius).
- Each chicken breast should have a pocket cut into it.
- Cherry tomatoes, mozzarella cheese, and chopped basil should be stuffed into each chicken breast filling.
- Use salt and black pepper to season the food.
- Prepare the olive oil by heating it in a pan over medium-high heat.
- Chicken breasts should be browned for two to three minutes on each side.
- Place the chicken in a baking dish and bake it for twenty to twenty-five minutes, or until it is completely cooked through.
- Apply a glaze made with balsamic vinegar just before serving.

Nutritional Value (per serving):

- Calories: 260
- Protein: 41g
- Carbohydrates: 5g
- Fiber: 3g
- Healthy fats: 10g

Mediterranean Chickpea and Quinoa Salad

Ingredients:

- 1 cup cooked quinoa
- 1 can (15 oz) chickpeas, drained and rinsed
- 1 cup diced cucumber
- 1 cup cherry tomatoes, halved
- 1/2 cup diced red onion
- 1/4 cup Kalamata olives, pitted and sliced
- Feta cheese (optional)
- Greek dressing

Instructions:

- Combine the quinoa that has been cooked, the chickpeas, the cucumber, the cherry tomatoes, the red onion, and the Kalamata olives in a bowl.
- After drizzling with Greek dressing, stir the ingredients together.
- Crumbled feta cheese may be sprinkled on top if desired.

Nutritional Value (per serving):

- Calories: 322
- Protein: 11g
- Carbohydrates: 52g
- Fiber: 13g
- Healthy fats: 10g

Lemon Garlic Butter Shrimp Pasta

Ingredients:

- 8 oz (226g) whole wheat pasta
- 1 lb (450g) shrimp, peeled and deveined
- Zest and juice of 1 lemon
- 2 cloves garlic, minced
- 2 tablespoons unsalted butter
- Fresh parsley for garnish Salt and black pepper to taste

Instructions:

- Cook the pasta following the directions on the package. Drain, then keep away for later use.
- Over medium-high heat, butter should be melted in a small pan.
- Sauté the garlic that has been minced for one to two minutes.
- Make sure the shrimp are pink and opaque before adding them.
- The lemon zest, lemon juice, cooked pasta, salt, and black pepper should be stirred in at this point.
- Immediately before serving, garnish with fresh parsley.

Nutritional Value (per serving):

- Calories: 383
- Protein: 36g
- Carbohydrates: 49g

- Fiber: 8g

- Healthy fats: 10g

Thai Vegetable Curry

Ingredients:

- 2 cups mixed vegetables (e.g., bell peppers, zucchini, carrots)
- 1 can (15 oz) coconut milk
- 2 tablespoons Thai red curry paste
- 1 tablespoon vegetable oil
- 1 tablespoon soy sauce
- Cooked jasmine rice

Instructions:

- Oil made from vegetables should be heated in a large pan over medium-high heat.
- Add a variety of veggies and stir-fry them for three to five minutes.
- The Thai red curry paste should be stirred in and cooked for two minutes.
- Add the soy sauce and coconut milk to the mixture. Simmer for five to seven minutes.
- Serve over cooked jasmine rice.

Nutritional Value (per serving):

- Calories: 359
- Protein: 7g
- Carbohydrates: 12g
- Fiber: 6g
- Healthy fats: 33g

Grilled Vegetable and Quinoa Salad

Ingredients:

- 1 cup cooked quinoa
- 2 cups mixed grilled vegetables (e.g., eggplant, zucchini, bell peppers)
- 1/4 cup crumbled feta cheese
- 2 tablespoons balsamic vinaigrette
- Fresh basil leaves for garnish Salt and black pepper to taste

Instructions:

- Mixed veggies should be grilled until they are soft and have a little char.
- Quinoa that has been cooked, veggies that have been grilled, crumbled feta cheese, balsamic vinaigrette, salt, and black pepper should be mixed in a bowl.
- Before serving, garnish with fresh basil leaves from the garden.

Nutritional Value (per serving):

- Calories: 287
- Protein: 9g
- Carbohydrates: 32g
- Fiber: 7g
- Healthy fats: 13g

Beef and Vegetable Skewers

Ingredients:

- 1 lb (450g) beef sirloin, cut into cubes
- 2 cups mixed vegetables (e.g., cherry tomatoes, bell peppers, mushrooms)
- 2 tablespoons olive oil
- 2 cloves garlic, minced
- 1 tablespoon Italian seasoning
- Wooden skewers, soaked in water

Instructions:

- Olive oil, garlic that has been minced, and Italian spice should be mixed in a basin.
- Use wooden skewers to thread beef pieces and a variety of veggies onto the skewers.
- Apply the olive oil mixture on the skewers and brush them.

- Skewers should be grilled over medium-high heat for eight to ten minutes, flipping them regularly, until the meat reaches the desired level of doneness.
- Serve with a side salad or rice.

Nutritional Value (per serving):

- Calories: 324
- Protein: 33g
- Carbohydrates: 11g
- Fiber: 3g
- Healthy fats: 19g

Stuffed Acorn Squash

Ingredients:

- 2 acorn squash, halved and seeds removed
- 1 cup quinoa, cooked
- 1/2 cup dried cranberries
- 1/4 cup chopped pecans
- 2 tablespoons maple syrup
- Cinnamon for sprinkling
- Olive oil for brushing

Instructions:

- Preheat the oven to 375 degrees Fahrenheit (190 degrees Celsius).

- Olive oil should be used to coat the sliced sides of the acorn squash, and cinnamon should be sprinkled on top.

- To roast squash halves, place them on a baking sheet with the cut side down. Roast them for thirty to forty minutes, or until they are soft.

- Combine quinoa that has been cooked, dried cranberries, pecans that have been chopped, and maple syrup in a bowl.

- The quinoa mixture should be stuffed into each side of the acorn squash.

- Keep baking for a further ten to fifteen minutes.

- Both a lovely side dish and a light dinner option, serve this meal.

Nutritional Value (per serving, 1 stuffed squash half):

- Calories: 323

- Protein: 7g

- Carbohydrates: 62g

- Fiber: 9g

- Healthy fats: 9g

DESSERT RECIPES

Greek Yogurt Parfait

Ingredients:

- 1/2 cup Greek yogurt
- 1/4 cup mixed berries (e.g., strawberries, blueberries)
- 2 tablespoons granola
- 1 teaspoon honey (optional)

Instructions:

- Greek yogurt, mixed berries, and granola should be layered side by side in a dish or glass.
- You may drizzle honey on top if you want.

Nutritional Value (per serving):

- Calories: 202
- Protein: 11g
- Carbohydrates: 34g
- Fiber: 6g
- Healthy fats: 6g

Chocolate Banana Chia Pudding

Ingredients:

- 2 tablespoons chia seeds

- 1 cup almond milk (or any milk of your choice)

- 1 ripe banana, mashed

- 1 tablespoon cocoa powder

- 1/2 teaspoon vanilla extract

Instructions:

- Chia seeds, almond milk, mashed banana, chocolate powder, and vanilla essence should be mixed in a bowl or any other container. Give it a good stir.

- Cover and place in the refrigerator for the night.

- Give it a nice stir in the morning, and then take pleasure in it.

Nutritional Value (per serving):

- Calories: 210

- Protein: 5g

- Carbohydrates: 36g

- Fiber: 11g

- Healthy fats: 7g

Mixed Berry Smoothie Bowl

Ingredients:

- 1 cup mixed berries (e.g., strawberries, blueberries, raspberries)

- 1/2 banana

- 1/2 cup Greek yogurt

- 1/4 cup granola

- 1 tablespoon almond butter

Instructions:

- Mix the mixed berries, banana, and Greek yogurt in a blender until the mixture is completely smooth.

- The smoothie should be poured into a bowl.

- Nut butter and granola should be sprinkled over top.

Nutritional Value (per serving):

- Calories: 282

- Protein: 16g

- Carbohydrates: 46g

- Fiber: 12g

- Healthy fats: 9g

Apple Cinnamon Baked Oatmeal Cups

Ingredients:

- 1 cup rolled oats

- 1/2 cup unsweetened applesauce

- 1/4 cup milk of your choice

- 1 egg

- 1 teaspoon cinnamon

- 1/2 teaspoon vanilla extract

- 1 apple, diced

Instructions:

- Prepare a muffin tray by greasing it and preheating the oven to 350 degrees Fahrenheit (175 degrees Celsius).

- Oats that have been rolled, applesauce, milk, an egg, cinnamon, and vanilla essence should be combined in a bowl.

- Mix in the apple that has been diced.

- Place a little of the mixture in each of the muffin cups.

- Bake for twenty to twenty-five minutes, or until the mixture is firm and golden brown.

Nutritional Value (per serving - 2 oatmeal cups):

- Calories: 253

- Protein: 9g

- Carbohydrates: 44g

- Fiber: 4g

- Healthy fats: 6g

Peanut Butter Banana Ice Cream

Ingredients:

- 2 ripe bananas, sliced and frozen

- 2 tablespoons peanut butter

- 1 tablespoon cocoa powder (optional)

Instructions:

- Using a blender or food processor, place frozen banana slices in the container.
- If you are using cocoa powder and peanut butter, add them now.
- Blend until it is completely smooth and creamy, stopping to scrape down the sides as necessary.
- If you want a more firm texture, you may freeze it or serve it immediately as soft-serve.

Nutritional Value (per serving):

- Calories: 283
- Protein: 6g
- Carbohydrates: 44g
- Fiber: 7g
- Healthy fats: 13g

Almond Butter Energy Bites

Ingredients:

- 1 cup old-fashioned oats
- 1/2 cup almond butter
- 1/4 cup honey
- 1/4 cup chopped almonds

- 1/4 cup dark chocolate chips

- 1 teaspoon vanilla extract

- Pinch of salt

Instructions:

- Oats, almond butter, honey, chopped almonds, chocolate chips, vanilla essence, and a bit of salt should be mixed in a bowl after being combined.

- After thoroughly combining, mix.

- To make bite-sized balls, roll the mixture into chunks.

- The dish should be chilled for at least half an hour before being consumed.

Nutritional Value (per serving - 2 energy bites):

- Calories: 221

- Protein: 5g

- Carbohydrates: 24g

- Fiber: 5g

- Healthy fats: 10g

Strawberry Banana Frozen Yogurt

Ingredients:

- 2 cups frozen strawberries

- 2 ripe bananas

- 1/2 cup Greek yogurt 1 tablespoon honey (optional)

Instructions:

- Honey, frozen strawberries, and bananas should be placed in a blender. Greek yogurt can also be added.
- Puree till it is silky smooth and creamy.
- If you want a more firm texture, you may freeze it or serve it immediately as soft-serve.

Nutritional Value (per serving):

- Calories: 182
- Protein: 7g
- Carbohydrates: 39g
- Fiber: 7g
- Healthy fats: 2g

Oatmeal Raisin Cookies

Ingredients:

- 1 cup old-fashioned oats
- 1/2 cup whole wheat flour
- 1/4 cup raisins
- 1/4 cup chopped walnuts
- 1/4 cup honey
- 1/4 cup unsweetened applesauce
- 1 egg
- 1 teaspoon cinnamon

- 1/2 teaspoon vanilla extract

Instructions:

- Line a baking sheet with parchment paper and preheat the oven to 175 degrees Celsius (350 degrees Fahrenheit).
- Oats, whole wheat flour, raisins, chopped walnuts, honey, applesauce, egg, cinnamon, and vanilla extract should be combined in a bowl and then stirred together.
- To flatten the dough somewhat, drop spoonfuls of it onto the baking sheet and then flatten it.
- To get a golden brown color, bake for 12 to 15 minutes.

Nutritional Value (per serving - 2 cookies):

- Calories: 219
- Protein: 8g
- Carbohydrates: 31g
- Fiber: 5g
- Healthy fats: 6g

Chocolate Avocado Mousse

Ingredients:

- 2 ripe avocados
- 1/4 cup unsweetened cocoa powder
- 1/4 cup honey or maple syrup
- 1 teaspoon vanilla extract

- Pinch of salt
- Berries for topping

Instructions:

- Avocados, cocoa powder, honey or maple syrup, vanilla essence, and a sprinkling of salt should be blended in a food processor until the mixture is completely smooth.
- Create individual serving cups out of the mousse.
- At least one hour should be spent chilling the dish in the refrigerator before served.
- Before you taste it, garnish it with berries.

Nutritional Value (per serving):

- Calories: 210
- Protein: 4g
- Carbohydrates: 27g
- Fiber: 9g
- Healthy fats: 13g

Rice Pudding with Cinnamon

Ingredients:

- 1/2 cup cooked white rice
- 1 cup milk of your choice
- 2 tablespoons honey or maple syrup
- 1/2 teaspoon vanilla extract

- 1/2 teaspoon cinnamon
- Raisins or chopped nuts for topping

Instructions:

- The rice that has been cooked, milk, honey or maple syrup, vanilla essence, and cinnamon should be mixed in a saucepan.
- Over medium heat, bring to a simmer, and continue cooking while stirring constantly until the mixture has thickened.
- Take it off the heat and let it cool down a little bit.
- Place raisins or chopped nuts on top of the dish and serve either warm or cooled.

Nutritional Value (per serving):

- Calories: 253
- Protein: 7g
- Carbohydrates: 42g
- Fiber: 2g
- Healthy fats: 7g

Fruit Salad with Honey-Lime Drizzle

Ingredients:

- 1 cup mixed fruits (e.g., pineapple chunks, melon, grapes, berries)
- 1 tablespoon honey

- Juice of 1 lime

- Fresh mint leaves for garnish

Instructions:

- Blend a variety of fruits in a dish.

- Honey and lime juice should be mixed in a small bowl using a whisk.

- To finish off the fruit salad, drizzle the honey-lime mixture over it.

- Include some fresh mint leaves as a garnish.

Nutritional Value (per serving):

- Calories: 83

- Protein: 2g

- Carbohydrates: 22g

- Fiber: 2g

- Healthy fats: 0g

Baked Apples with Cinnamon and Walnuts

Ingredients:

- 2 apples, cored and halved

- 2 tablespoons chopped walnuts

- 1 teaspoon cinnamon

- 1 tablespoon honey

- Greek yogurt for topping (optional)

Instructions:

- Using parchment paper, line a baking dish and preheat the oven to 350 degrees Fahrenheit (175 degrees Celsius).

- Apple halves should be placed in the dish.

- Chop the walnuts and combine them with the cinnamon and honey in a bowl.

- Dollop the walnut mixture into the apple halves using a spoon.

- Bake for twenty to twenty-five minutes, or until the apples are soft.

- Depending on your preference, serve with a dollop of Greek yogurt.

Nutritional Value (per serving - 1 apple half):

- Calories: 111

- Protein: 3g

- Carbohydrates: 22g

- Fiber: 5g

- Healthy fats: 5g

Blueberry Almond Smoothie

Ingredients:

- 1/2 cup frozen blueberries

- 1/2 banana

- 1 cup almond milk (or any milk of your choice)
- 2 tablespoons almond butter
- 1 tablespoon honey

Instructions:

- Blueberries that have been frozen, banana, almond milk, almond butter, and honey should be blended in a blender.
- Blend until it is completely smooth.
- To enjoy, pour the mixture into a glass.

Nutritional Value (per serving):

- Calories: 292
- Protein: 7g
- Carbohydrates: 42g
- Fiber: 7g
- Healthy fats: 14g

Chia Seed Chocolate Pudding

Ingredients:

- 2 tablespoons chia seeds
- 1 cup almond milk (or any milk of your choice)
- 1 tablespoon unsweetened cocoa powder
- 1 tablespoon honey or maple syrup
- 1/2 teaspoon vanilla extract

Instructions:

- In a jar or dish, mix the chia seeds, almond milk, chocolate powder, honey or maple syrup, and vanilla extract. Stir thoroughly.
- Cover and refrigerate for at least 3 hours or overnight.
- Stir before serving. If preferred, add a little more milk.

Nutritional Value (per serving):

- Calories: 182
- Protein: 5g
- Carbohydrates: 23g
- Fiber: 10g
- Healthy fats: 11g

Mixed Nut and Berry Bars

Ingredients:

- 1 cup mixed nuts (e.g., almonds, cashews, walnuts)
- 1/2 cup dried berries (e.g., cranberries, blueberries)
- 1/4 cup honey
- 1/4 cup almond butter
- 1/2 teaspoon vanilla extract
- Pinch of salt

Instructions:

- The mixed nuts should be pulsed in a food processor until they are coarsely minced.

- Mix in some honey, almond butter, vanilla essence, and dried berries, and then season with a little bit of salt. Pulse until everything is well blended.

- In a square baking pan that has been lined, press the ingredients gently.

- After letting it chill for at least two hours, chop it into bars.

Nutritional Value (per serving - 1 bar):

- Calories: 220

- Protein: 5g

- Carbohydrates: 19g

- Fiber: 4g

- Healthy fats: 14g

No-Bake Energy Bars

Ingredients:

- 1 cup rolled oats

- 1/2 cup almond butter

- 1/4 cup honey

- 1/4 cup chopped dried fruits (e.g., apricots, dates)

- 1/4 cup chopped nuts (e.g., almonds, cashews)

- 1/4 cup dark chocolate chips

- 1/2 teaspoon vanilla extract

- In a bowl, combine rolled oats, almond butter, honey, dried fruits, chopped nuts, dark chocolate chips, and vanilla extract.
- Mix until well combined.
- Press the mixture into a lined square baking pan.
- Refrigerate for at least 2 hours, then cut into bars.

Nutritional Value (per serving - 1 bar):

- Calories: 242
- Protein: 7g
- Carbohydrates: 25g
- Fiber: 6g
- Healthy fats: 14g

Mango Sorbet

Ingredients:

- 2 ripe mangoes, peeled and diced
- 2 tablespoons honey or maple syrup
- Juice of 1 lime

Instructions:

- The mangoes should be sliced, honey or maple syrup should be added, and lime juice should be blended.
- The mixture should be smooth.

- After pouring into a container, freeze the mixture for at least four hours, stirring it every hour until it becomes hard.

- A dollop of mango sorbet should be served.

Nutritional Value (per serving):

- Calories: 123

- Protein: 2g

- Carbohydrates: 33g

- Fiber: 4g

- Healthy fats: 0g

Cinnamon Roasted Almonds

Ingredients:

- 1 cup raw almonds

- 1 tablespoon honey

- 1 teaspoon ground cinnamon

- Pinch of salt

Instructions:

- Line a baking sheet with parchment paper and preheat the oven to 175 degrees Celsius (350 degrees Fahrenheit).

- To prepare the raw almonds, combine them in a dish with honey, ground cinnamon, and a little bit of salt.

- The almonds should be distributed equally throughout the baking sheet.

- Roast for ten to fifteen minutes, stirring halfway through, until the aroma is released and the toastiness is heightened.
- First, let them cool down before serving.

Nutritional Value (per serving - 1/4 cup):

- Calories: 182
- Protein: 6g
- Carbohydrates: 10g
- Fiber: 4g
- Healthy fats: 12g

Pumpkin Pie Smoothie

Ingredients:

- 1/2 cup canned pumpkin puree
- 1/2 banana
- 1 cup almond milk (or any milk of your choice)
- 1/2 teaspoon pumpkin pie spice
- 1 tablespoon honey or maple syrup
- Ice cubes

Instructions:

- In a blender, combine pumpkin puree, banana, almond milk, pumpkin pie spice, honey or maple syrup, and ice cubes.
- Blend until smooth.

- Pour into a glass and sprinkle with extra pumpkin pie spice if desired.

Nutritional Value (per serving):

- Calories: 182
- Protein: 3g
- Carbohydrates: 39g
- Fiber: 6g
- Healthy fats: 5g

Chocolate-Dipped Strawberries

Ingredients:

- 10 fresh strawberries, rinsed and dried
- 1/4 cup dark chocolate chips
- 1/2 teaspoon coconut oil

Instructions:

- In a microwave-safe bowl, melt dark chocolate chips and coconut oil in 20-second intervals, stirring in between, until smooth.
- Dip each strawberry into the melted chocolate, covering half or two-thirds of the berry.
- Place on a parchment-lined tray.
- Refrigerate until the chocolate hardens.
- Enjoy your chocolate-dipped strawberries!

Nutritional Value (per serving - 2 strawberries):

- Calories: 102
- Protein: 3g
- Carbohydrates: 16g
- Fiber: 3g
- Healthy fats: 6g

Berry and Greek Yogurt Popsicles

Ingredients:

- 1 cup mixed berries (e.g., strawberries, blueberries, raspberries)
- 1 cup Greek yogurt
- 2 tablespoons honey
- Popsicle molds or small cups and popsicle sticks

Instructions:

- Melt the honey, Greek yogurt, and mixed berries together in a blender until they are completely smooth.
- If you have popsicle molds or little cups, pour the mixture into them.
- Popsicle sticks should be inserted into the middle.
- Put in the freezer for at least four hours, or until it becomes solid.

Nutritional Value (per serving):

- Calories: 92
- Protein: 7g
- Carbohydrates: 16g
- Fiber: 4g
- Healthy fats: 2g

Peanut Butter Banana Oat Cookies

Ingredients:

- 2 ripe bananas, mashed
- 1 cup old-fashioned oats
- 1/4 cup peanut butter
- 1/4 cup dark chocolate chips (optional)
- 1/2 teaspoon vanilla extract

Instructions:

- Line a baking sheet with parchment paper and preheat the oven to 175 degrees Celsius (350 degrees Fahrenheit).
- Put the mashed bananas, oats, peanut butter, dark chocolate chips, and vanilla essence into a bowl and mix this mixture.
- To flatten the dough somewhat, drop spoonfuls of it onto the baking sheet and then flatten it.
- To get a golden brown color, bake for 12 to 15 minutes.

Nutritional Value (per serving - 2 cookies):

- Calories: 210

- Protein: 7g

- Carbohydrates: 32g

- Fiber: 5g

- Healthy fats: 9g

Watermelon and Mint Granita

Ingredients:

- 4 cups cubed seedless watermelon

- 2 tablespoons fresh lime juice

- 1 tablespoon honey (optional)

- Fresh mint leaves for garnish

Instructions:

- Mix the watermelon, lime juice, and honey in a blender until the mixture is completely smooth.

- Using a shallow dish, pour the mixture into the dish.

- For about one hour, or when it begins to freeze around the edges, place it in the freezer.

- The ice edges should be scraped with a fork and then mixed into the middle of the mixture.

- This procedure should be repeated every half an hour for about two to three hours, or until the whole mixture has become ice and granular.

- Serve with fresh mint leaves.

Nutritional Value (per serving):

- Calories: 61
- Protein: 2g
- Carbohydrates: 16g
- Fiber: 4g
- Healthy fats: 0g

Avocado Chocolate Mousse

Ingredients:

- 2 ripe avocados
- 1/4 cup unsweetened cocoa powder
- 1/4 cup honey or maple syrup
- 1/2 teaspoon vanilla extract
- Pinch of salt
- Fresh berries for topping

Instructions:

- Avocados, cocoa powder, honey or maple syrup, vanilla essence, and a sprinkling of salt should be blended in a food processor until the mixture is completely smooth.
- Create individual serving cups out of the mousse.
- At least one hour should be spent chilling the dish in the refrigerator before served.
- Before you taste it, garnish it with some fresh berries.

Nutritional Value (per serving):

- Calories: 198
- Protein: 4g
- Carbohydrates: 26g
- Fiber: 9g
- Healthy fats: 11g

Almond and Coconut Energy Balls

Ingredients:

- 1 cup almonds
- 1/2 cup shredded coconut
- 1/4 cup honey or maple syrup
- 1/4 cup almond butter
- 1/2 teaspoon vanilla extract
- Pinch of salt

Instructions:

- In a food processor, pulse almonds until finely chopped.
- Combine shredded coconut, honey or maple syrup, almond butter, vanilla essence, and a bit of salt.
- Pulse until well blended.
- Roll the mixture into bite-sized balls.
- Refrigerate for a minimum of 30 minutes before serving.

Nutritional Value (per serving - 2 energy balls):

- Calories: 183
- Protein: 5g
- Carbohydrates: 19g
- Fiber: 4g
- Healthy fats: 13g

SOUP RECIPES

Turmeric Lentil Soup

Ingredients:

- 1 cup dried red lentils
- 1 onion, chopped
- 2 carrots, diced
- 2 celery stalks, chopped
- 3 cloves garlic, minced
- 1 teaspoon turmeric powder
- 1 teaspoon cumin
- 6 cups vegetable broth
- Salt and pepper to taste
- Fresh cilantro for garnish

Instructions:

- Rinse lentils under cold water.
- In a large pot, sauté onion, carrots, and celery until softened.
- Add minced garlic, turmeric, and cumin, stirring for 1-2 minutes.
- Pour in vegetable broth and add lentils. Bring to a boil, then simmer for 20-25 minutes.

- Season with salt and pepper. Garnish with fresh cilantro before serving.

Nutritional Information:

- Calories: 220
- Protein: 15g
- Fat: 1g
- Carbohydrates: 40g
- Fiber: 15g

Roasted Tomato Basil Soup

Ingredients:

- 8 tomatoes, halved
- 1 onion, quartered
- 4 cloves garlic, peeled
- 2 tablespoons olive oil
- 4 cups vegetable broth
- 1 cup fresh basil leaves
- Salt and pepper to taste
- 1/4 cup grated Parmesan cheese (optional)

Instructions:

- Preheat the oven to 400°F (200°C).
- Place tomatoes, onion, and garlic on a baking sheet. Drizzle with olive oil and roast for 30 minutes.

- Transfer roasted vegetables to a pot. Add vegetable broth and simmer for 15 minutes.
- Blend the mixture with fresh basil until smooth.
- Season with salt and pepper. Top with Parmesan if desired.

Nutritional Information:

- Calories: 180
- Protein: 5g
- Fat: 9g
- Carbohydrates: 22g
- Fiber: 6g

Spicy Black Bean Soup

Ingredients:

- 2 cans (15 oz each) of black beans, drained and rinsed
- 1 onion, diced
- 1 bell pepper, chopped
- 2 cloves garlic, minced
- 1 teaspoon cumin
- 1/2 teaspoon chili powder
- 4 cups vegetable broth
- 1 cup corn kernels
- Fresh cilantro for garnish
- Lime wedges for serving

Instructions:

- In a pot, sauté onion, bell pepper, and garlic until softened.
- Add cumin and chili powder, stirring for 1-2 minutes.
- Pour in vegetable broth, add black beans, and bring to a simmer for 15 minutes.
- Add corn and cook for an additional 5 minutes.
- Garnish with fresh cilantro and serve with lime wedges.

Nutritional Information:

- Calories: 250
- Protein: 12g
- Fat: 1g
- Carbohydrates: 50g
- Fiber: 15g

Coconut Curry Butternut Squash Soup

Ingredients:

- 1 butternut squash, peeled and diced
- 1 onion, chopped
- 2 tablespoons curry powder
- 1 can (14 oz) coconut milk
- 4 cups vegetable broth
- 1 tablespoon olive oil
- Salt and pepper to taste

- Chopped cilantro for garnish

Instructions:

- In a large pot, sauté onion in olive oil until translucent.
- Add curry powder and diced butternut squash, stirring for 3-5 minutes.
- Pour in vegetable broth and bring to a boil. Simmer until the squash is tender.
- Blend the soup with coconut milk until smooth.
- Season with salt and pepper. Garnish with chopped cilantro.

Nutritional Information:

- Calories: 280
- Protein: 5g
- Fat: 20g
- Carbohydrates: 25g
- Fiber: 5g

Mushroom and Barley Soup

Ingredients:

- 1 cup pearl barley
- 8 oz mushrooms, sliced
- 1 onion, diced
- 2 carrots, sliced
- 2 celery stalks, chopped

- 4 cups vegetable broth

- 2 cloves garlic, minced

- 1 teaspoon thyme

- Salt and pepper to taste

Instructions:

- Cook pearl barley according to package instructions.

- In a pot, sauté mushrooms, onion, carrots, and celery until softened.

- Add minced garlic and thyme, stirring for 1-2 minutes.

- Pour in vegetable broth and add cooked barley. Simmer for 15-20 minutes.

- Season with salt and pepper before serving.

Nutritional Information:

- Calories: 230

- Protein: 8g

- Fat: 1g

- Carbohydrates: 50g

- Fiber: 10g

Tuscan White Bean and Kale Soup

Ingredients:

- 2 cans (15 oz each) white beans, drained and rinsed

- 1 bunch of kale, stems removed and chopped

- 1 onion, chopped
- 3 cloves garlic, minced
- 1 can (14 oz) diced tomatoes
- 4 cups vegetable broth
- 2 tablespoons olive oil
- 1 teaspoon rosemary
- Salt and pepper to taste

Instructions:

- In a pot, sauté onion in olive oil until softened.
- Add minced garlic, chopped kale, and rosemary, stirring until kale wilts.
- Pour in vegetable broth, add white beans and diced tomatoes. Simmer for 15-20 minutes.
- Season with salt and pepper before serving.

Nutritional Information:

- Calories: 260
- Protein: 12g
- Fat: 5g
- Carbohydrates: 45g
- Fiber: 12g

Chicken and Vegetable Quinoa Soup

Ingredients:

- 1 cup cooked quinoa
- 2 chicken breasts, cooked and shredded
- 2 carrots, sliced
- 2 celery stalks, chopped
- 1 onion, diced
- 4 cups chicken broth
- 2 cloves garlic, minced
- 1 teaspoon thyme
- Salt and pepper to taste

Instructions:

- In a pot, sauté onion, carrots, and celery until softened.
- Add minced garlic and shredded chicken, stirring for 2-3 minutes.
- Pour in chicken broth and bring to a simmer. Add cooked quinoa.
- Season with thyme, salt, and pepper. Simmer for an additional 15 minutes.

Nutritional Information:

- Calories: 320
- Protein: 25g
- Fat: 5g

- Carbohydrates: 40g

- Fiber: 6g

Spinach and Chickpea Soup

Ingredients:

- 1 can (15 oz) chickpeas, drained and rinsed

- 4 cups fresh spinach

- 1 onion, chopped

- 2 carrots, diced

- 2 cloves garlic, minced

- 4 cups vegetable broth

- 2 tablespoons olive oil

- 1 teaspoon cumin

- Salt and pepper to taste

Instructions:

- In a pot, sauté onion, carrots, and garlic in olive oil until softened.

- Add chickpeas and cumin, stirring for 2-3 minutes.

- Pour in vegetable broth and bring to a simmer. Add fresh spinach.

- Simmer until spinach wilts. Season with salt and pepper before serving.

Nutritional Information:

- Calories: 250

- Protein: 10g

- Fat: 8g

- Carbohydrates: 40g

- Fiber: 10g

Sweet Potato and Ginger Soup

Ingredients:

- 2 large sweet potatoes, peeled and diced

- 1 onion, chopped

- 2 tablespoons fresh ginger, grated

- 4 cups vegetable broth

- 1 can (14 oz) coconut milk

- 2 tablespoons olive oil

- Salt and pepper to taste

Instructions:

- In a pot, sauté onion in olive oil until translucent.

- Add diced sweet potatoes and grated ginger, stirring for 3-4 minutes.

- Pour in vegetable broth and bring to a boil. Simmer until sweet potatoes are tender.

- Blend the soup with coconut milk until smooth. Season with salt and pepper.

Nutritional Information:

- Calories: 290
- Protein: 5g
- Fat: 12g
- Carbohydrates: 40g
- Fiber: 8g

Cauliflower and Leek Soup

Ingredients:

- 1 cauliflower, chopped
- 2 leeks, sliced
- 3 cloves garlic, minced
- 4 cups vegetable broth
- 1/2 cup almond milk
- 2 tablespoons olive oil
- 1 teaspoon thyme
- Salt and pepper to taste

Instructions:

- In a pot, sauté leeks and garlic in olive oil until softened.
- Add chopped cauliflower and thyme, stirring for 3-4 minutes.

- Pour in vegetable broth and bring to a simmer. Cook until cauliflower is tender.
- Blend the soup with almond milk until creamy. Season with salt and pepper.

Nutritional Information:

- Calories: 210
- Protein: 5g
- Fat: 10g
- Carbohydrates: 30g
- Fiber: 10g

VEGETARIAN RECIPES

Quinoa-Stuffed Bell Peppers

Ingredients:

- 4 bell peppers, halved
- 1 cup quinoa, cooked
- 1 can (15 oz) black beans, drained and rinsed
- 1 cup corn kernels
- 1 cup cherry tomatoes, halved
- 1 teaspoon cumin
- 1/2 teaspoon chili powder
- Salt and pepper to taste
- Fresh cilantro for garnish

Instructions:

- Preheat the oven to 375°F (190°C).
- In a bowl, mix cooked quinoa, black beans, corn, cherry tomatoes, cumin, chili powder, salt, and pepper.
- Stuff bell pepper halves with the quinoa mixture.
- Bake for 25-30 minutes until peppers are tender.
- Garnish with fresh cilantro before serving.

Nutritional Information:

- Calories: 220

- Protein: 10g

- Fat: 2g

- Carbohydrates: 45g

- Fiber: 8g

Chickpea and Spinach Curry

Ingredients:

- 2 cans (15 oz each) chickpeas, drained and rinsed

- 1 onion, chopped

- 2 tomatoes, diced

- 3 cups fresh spinach

- 2 cloves garlic, minced

- 1 tablespoon curry powder

- 1 can (14 oz) coconut milk

- 2 tablespoons olive oil

- Salt and pepper to taste

Instructions:

- In a pan, sauté chopped onion and minced garlic in olive oil until softened.

- Add chickpeas, diced tomatoes, and curry powder, stirring for 3-4 minutes.

- Pour in coconut milk and simmer until the sauce thickens.

- Add fresh spinach and cook until wilted.

- Season with salt and pepper before serving.

Nutritional Information:

- Calories: 280
- Protein: 10g
- Fat: 14g
- Carbohydrates: 30g
- Fiber: 10g

Eggplant Parmesan

Ingredients:

- 2 large eggplants, sliced
- 2 cups marinara sauce
- 1 cup breadcrumbs
- 1 cup grated Parmesan cheese
- 2 cups mozzarella cheese, shredded
- 2 tablespoons olive oil
- 1 teaspoon dried oregano
- Salt and pepper to taste

Instructions:

- Preheat the oven to 375°F (190°C).
- Brush eggplant slices with olive oil and season with salt and pepper.
- Coat each slice in breadcrumbs and arrange in a baking dish.

- Pour marinara sauce over the eggplant. Top with mozzarella and Parmesan.

- Bake for 30-35 minutes until cheese is melted and bubbly.

- Sprinkle dried oregano before serving.

Nutritional Information:

- Calories: 320

- Protein: 15g

- Fat: 15g

- Carbohydrates: 35g

- Fiber: 8g

Sweet Potato and Black Bean Tacos

Ingredients:

- 8 small corn tortillas

- 2 sweet potatoes, diced

- 1 can (15 oz) black beans, drained and rinsed

- 1 avocado, sliced

- 1 cup shredded lettuce

- 1/2 cup diced red onion

- 1 teaspoon cumin

- 1/2 teaspoon paprika

- 2 tablespoons olive oil

- Fresh cilantro for garnish

Instructions:

- Toss diced sweet potatoes with cumin, paprika, and olive oil. Roast until tender.
- Warm corn tortillas in a pan.
- Assemble tacos with roasted sweet potatoes, black beans, avocado, lettuce, and red onion.
- Garnish with fresh cilantro before serving.

Nutritional Information:

- Calories: 250
- Protein: 8g
- Fat: 10g
- Carbohydrates: 35g
- Fiber: 10g

Mushroom and Spinach Risotto

Ingredients:

- 2 cups Arborio rice
- 8 oz mushrooms, sliced
- 3 cups fresh spinach
- 1 onion, diced
- 4 cups vegetable broth
- 1 cup dry white wine
- 1/2 cup Parmesan cheese, grated

- 2 tablespoons olive oil
- Salt and pepper to taste

Instructions:

- In a pan, sauté diced onion in olive oil until translucent.
- Add Arborio rice and cook for 2-3 minutes.
- Pour in dry white wine and simmer until absorbed.
- Add vegetable broth gradually, stirring continuously until rice is creamy.
- Stir in sliced mushrooms and fresh spinach until wilted.
- Remove from heat, mix in Parmesan, and season with salt and pepper.

Nutritional Information:

- Calories: 300
- Protein: 8g
- Fat: 10g
- Carbohydrates: 40g
- Fiber: 6g

Zucchini Noodles with Pesto

Ingredients:

- 4 medium zucchinis, spiralized
- 1 cup cherry tomatoes, halved
- 1/2 cup pine nuts

- 1 cup fresh basil leaves

- 2 cloves garlic

- 1/2 cup Parmesan cheese, grated

- 1/2 cup olive oil

- Salt and pepper to taste

Instructions:

- Spiralize zucchini into noodles and set aside.

- In a blender, combine pine nuts, basil, garlic, Parmesan, salt, and pepper. Blend until smooth.

- While blending, slowly add olive oil until the pesto is well combined.

- Toss zucchini noodles with cherry tomatoes and pesto.

- Serve chilled or at room temperature.

Nutritional Information:

- Calories: 280

- Protein: 6g

- Fat: 25g

- Carbohydrates: 10g

- Fiber: 4g

Lentil and Vegetable Stir-Fry

Ingredients:

- 1 cup dry green lentils, cooked
- 1 broccoli head, florets only
- 2 bell peppers, sliced
- 1 carrot, julienned
- 1 cup snap peas
- 3 tablespoons soy sauce
- 1 tablespoon sesame oil
- 2 cloves garlic, minced
- 1 tablespoon ginger, grated

Instructions:

- In a wok or pan, sauté garlic and ginger in sesame oil until fragrant.
- Add broccoli, bell peppers, carrots, and snap peas. Stir-fry until vegetables are crisp-tender.
- Add cooked lentils and soy sauce. Toss until well combined and heated through.
- Serve immediately.

Nutritional Information:

- Calories: 280
- Protein: 18g
- Fat: 5g

- Carbohydrates: 45g

- Fiber: 14g

Caprese Stuffed Portobello Mushrooms

Ingredients:

- 4 large portobello mushrooms, stems removed

- 1 cup cherry tomatoes, diced

- 1 cup fresh mozzarella, diced

- 1/2 cup fresh basil, chopped

- 2 tablespoons balsamic glaze

- 2 tablespoons olive oil

- Salt and pepper to taste

Instructions:

- Preheat the oven to 375°F (190°C).

- Place portobello mushrooms on a baking sheet.

- In a bowl, mix cherry tomatoes, mozzarella, basil, olive oil, salt, and pepper.

- Stuff each mushroom with the caprese mixture.

- Bake for 20-25 minutes until mushrooms are tender.

- Drizzle with balsamic glaze before serving.

Nutritional Information:

- Calories: 230

- Protein: 12g

- Fat: 15g

- Carbohydrates: 15g

- Fiber: 4g

Chickpea and Sweet Potato Curry

Ingredients:

- 2 cans (15 oz each) chickpeas, drained and rinsed

- 2 sweet potatoes, peeled and diced

- 1 can (14 oz) coconut milk

- 1 onion, chopped

- 2 tablespoons curry powder

- 2 tablespoons olive oil

- Salt and pepper to taste

Instructions:

- In a pot, sauté chopped onion in olive oil until softened.

- Add diced sweet potatoes, chickpeas, and curry powder, stirring for 3-4 minutes.

- Pour in coconut milk and bring to a simmer. Cook until sweet potatoes are tender.

- Season with salt and pepper before serving.

Nutritional Information:

- Calories: 310

- Protein: 10g

- Fat: 10g

- Carbohydrates: 45g

- Fiber: 10g

Mediterranean Quinoa Salad

Ingredients:

- 2 cups cooked quinoa

- 1 cucumber, diced

- 1 cup cherry tomatoes, halved

- 1/2 cup Kalamata olives, sliced

- 1/2 cup feta cheese, crumbled

- 1/4 cup red onion, finely chopped

- 2 tablespoons olive oil

- 1 tablespoon red wine vinegar

- Salt and pepper to taste

Instructions:

- In a bowl, combine cooked quinoa, cucumber, cherry tomatoes, olives, feta, and red onion.

- Drizzle olive oil and red wine vinegar over the salad. Toss until well coated.

- Season with salt and pepper before serving.

Nutritional Information:

- Calories: 280

- Protein: 8g

- Fat: 14g

- Carbohydrates: 30g

- Fiber: 6g

30-DAY MEAL PLAN

Day 1:

- Breakfast: Quinoa-stuffed Bell Peppers
- Lunch: Lentil and Vegetable Stir-Fry
- Dinner: Chickpea and Spinach Curry

Day 2:

- Breakfast: Sweet Potato and Black Bean Tacos
- Lunch: Caprese Stuffed Portobello Mushrooms
- Dinner: Mushroom and Spinach Risotto

Day 3:

- Breakfast: Zucchini Noodles with Pesto
- Lunch: Mediterranean Quinoa Salad
- Dinner: Chickpea and Sweet Potato Curry

Day 4:

- Breakfast: Quinoa-stuffed Bell Peppers
- Lunch: Lentil and Vegetable Stir-Fry
- Dinner: Eggplant Parmesan

Day 5:

- Breakfast: Sweet Potato and Black Bean Tacos
- Lunch: Caprese Stuffed Portobello Mushrooms

- Dinner: Zucchini Noodles with Pesto

Day 6:

- Breakfast: Mushroom and Spinach Risotto
- Lunch: Chickpea and Spinach Curry
- Dinner: Mediterranean Quinoa Salad

Day 7:

- Breakfast: Chickpea and Sweet Potato Curry
- Lunch: Lentil and Vegetable Stir-Fry
- Dinner: Sweet Potato and Black Bean Tacos

Day 8:

- Breakfast: Mushroom and Spinach Risotto
- Lunch: Chickpea and Sweet Potato Curry
- Dinner: Caprese Stuffed Portobello Mushrooms

Day 9:

- Breakfast: Zucchini Noodles with Pesto
- Lunch: Mediterranean Quinoa Salad
- Dinner: Lentil and Vegetable Stir-Fry

Day 10:

- Breakfast: Chickpea and Spinach Curry
- Lunch: Quinoa-stuffed Bell Peppers
- Dinner: Eggplant Parmesan

Day 11:

- Breakfast: Sweet Potato and Black Bean Tacos
- Lunch: Caprese Stuffed Portobello Mushrooms
- Dinner: Zucchini Noodles with Pesto

Day 12:

- Breakfast: Quinoa-stuffed Bell Peppers
- Lunch: Mediterranean Quinoa Salad
- Dinner: Chickpea and Spinach Curry

Day 13:

- Breakfast: Sweet Potato and Black Bean Tacos
- Lunch: Eggplant Parmesan
- Dinner: Lentil and Vegetable Stir-Fry

Day 14:

- Breakfast: Chickpea and Spinach Curry
- Lunch: Caprese Stuffed Portobello Mushrooms
- Dinner: Mushroom and Spinach Risotto

Day 15:

- Breakfast: Zucchini Noodles with Pesto
- Lunch: Sweet Potato and Black Bean Tacos
- Dinner: Quinoa-stuffed Bell Peppers

Day 16:

- Breakfast: Eggplant Parmesan
- Lunch: Mediterranean Quinoa Salad
- Dinner: Lentil and Vegetable Stir-Fry

Day 17:

- Breakfast: Chickpea and Sweet Potato Curry
- Lunch: Caprese Stuffed Portobello Mushrooms
- Dinner: Zucchini Noodles with Pesto

Day 18:

- Breakfast: Mushroom and Spinach Risotto
- Lunch: Quinoa-stuffed Bell Peppers
- Dinner: Eggplant Parmesan

Day 19:

- Breakfast: Sweet Potato and Black Bean Tacos
- Lunch: Mediterranean Quinoa Salad
- Dinner: Chickpea and Spinach Curry

Day 20:

- Breakfast: Zucchini Noodles with Pesto
- Lunch: Lentil and Vegetable Stir-Fry
- Dinner: Caprese Stuffed Portobello Mushrooms

Day 21:

- Breakfast: Chickpea and Spinach Curry
- Lunch: Sweet Potato and Black Bean Tacos
- Dinner: Mushroom and Spinach Risotto

Day 22:

- Breakfast: Quinoa-stuffed Bell Peppers
- Lunch: Caprese Stuffed Portobello Mushrooms
- Dinner: Sweet Potato and Black Bean Tacos

Day 23:

- Breakfast: Lentil and Vegetable Stir-Fry
- Lunch: Mediterranean Quinoa Salad
- Dinner: Mushroom and Spinach Risotto

Day 24:

- Breakfast: Zucchini Noodles with Pesto
- Lunch: Chickpea and Sweet Potato Curry
- Dinner: Eggplant Parmesan

Day 25:

- Breakfast: Caprese Stuffed Portobello Mushrooms
- Lunch: Quinoa-stuffed Bell Peppers
- Dinner: Sweet Potato and Black Bean Tacos

Day 26:

- Breakfast: Mediterranean Quinoa Salad
- Lunch: Mushroom and Spinach Risotto
- Dinner: Lentil and Vegetable Stir-Fry

Day 27:

- Breakfast: Sweet Potato and Black Bean Tacos
- Lunch: Chickpea and Spinach Curry
- Dinner: Zucchini Noodles with Pesto

Day 28:

- Breakfast: Eggplant Parmesan
- Lunch: Caprese Stuffed Portobello Mushrooms
- Dinner: Quinoa-stuffed Bell Peppers

Day 29:

- Breakfast: Zucchini Noodles with Pesto
- Lunch: Sweet Potato and Black Bean Tacos
- Dinner: Lentil and Vegetable Stir-Fry

Day 30:

- Breakfast: Chickpea and Spinach Curry
- Lunch: Quinoa-stuffed Bell Peppers
- Dinner: Mediterranean Quinoa Salad

Additional Tips:

- Stay hydrated by drinking plenty of water throughout the day.
- Snack on fresh fruits, nuts, or yogurt between meals if desired.
- Customize portions based on your individual dietary needs and activity levels.
- Listen to your body's hunger and fullness cues.